The Ileostomy Diet Cookbook

A Culinary Guide to Mastering the Ileostomy Diet and Living Your Best Life. Transform Your Post-Surgery Nutrition with Confidence and Creativity. Delicious Recipes for a Smooth and Happy Gut.

Harper Bloom

Copyright © 2024 Harper Bloom

Disclaimer: The information and recipes in this book are intended for general information purposes only and are not a substitute for professional medical advice. Always consult with your physician or qualified healthcare provider before making any dietary or lifestyle changes.

TABLE OF CONTENT

3 | The Ileostomy Diet Cookbook

Part 1: Introduction to the Ileostomy Diet

Introduction

A New Chapter, a Delicious Journey

Imagine a life filled with vibrant flavors, satisfying meals, and the freedom to explore a world of culinary delights. Now imagine this same life after ileostomy surgery. For many, the thought of an ileostomy can bring a wave of uncertainty, particularly when it comes to food. Can you still enjoy your favorite dishes? Will mealtimes become a constant struggle?

This book, "The Ileostomy Diet Cookbook: A Culinary Guide to Mastering the Ileostomy Diet and Living Your Best Life," is here to answer those questions with a resounding **yes!** We understand the challenges you face, because we've heard countless stories just like yours.

Juliet's Story:

Juliet, a vibrant young artist, had her world turned upside down when diagnosed with ulcerative colitis. After years of battling the disease, an ileostomy became her path forward.

"The thought of food restrictions terrified me," she recalls. "I loved spicy food, fresh salads, and everything in between. I couldn't imagine a life without those culinary adventures."

But Juliet wasn't alone. With the help of her doctor and a registered dietician, she learned to navigate the ileostomy diet. "It wasn't easy at first," she admits, "but this book became my lifesaver. I discovered delicious low-fibre recipes that were actually satisfying. Now, I can still enjoy social gatherings and create beautiful, healthy meals at home."

This is your story too.

"The Ileostomy Diet Cookbook" is more than just a collection of recipes. It's a roadmap to reclaiming your life and rediscovering the joy of food. We'll guide you through the fundamentals of the ileostomy diet, answer your burning questions, and equip you with the knowledge and confidence to create delicious, personalized meals.

Chapter 1: Mastering Your New Journey

Welcome to a Delicious New Chapter!

Imagine a life filled with flavorful dishes, satisfying meals, and the freedom to explore a world of culinary delights. Now imagine this same life thriving after ileostomy surgery. This book, "The Ileostomy Diet Cookbook," is your guide to reclaiming that freedom and proving that delicious food can still be a part of your story.

Understanding Your Ileostomy

An ileostomy is a surgical procedure that creates an opening (stoma) in your abdomen. The end of your small intestine (ileum) is brought out through this stoma, allowing waste to bypass the colon and rectum and exit into a collection pouch worn externally. This surgery is sometimes necessary for conditions like ulcerative colitis, Crohn's disease, or blockages in the colon.

Food as Fuel: Why Diet Matters After Ileostomy Surgery

Following ileostomy surgery, your digestive system works a little differently. The large intestine (colon) plays a vital role in absorbing water and electrolytes from waste. Without a colon, your body may have difficulty with this process, leading to dehydration and electrolyte imbalance.

The ileostomy diet focuses on keeping you feeling your best by:

- **Minimizing fibre intake:** High-fibre foods can be tricky for your small intestine to digest after surgery. We'll show you delicious low-fibre alternatives that won't compromise on flavor.

- **Staying Hydrated:** Drinking plenty of fluids is key to helping your body absorb nutrients and prevent dehydration. We'll provide tips and tricks to keep you hydrated throughout the day.

- **Maintaining a Balanced Plate:** Ensuring you get enough protein, vitamins, and minerals is crucial for overall health and healing. This book is packed with recipes that are as nutritious as they are tasty.

Challenges and Solutions: Conquering the Ileostomy Diet

While the ileostomy diet offers incredible benefits, it can also present some challenges:

- **Finding Flavorful Low-Fibre Options:** Many people enjoy the taste and texture of high-fibre foods. Don't worry, we've got you covered! This book is bursting with creative, low-fibre recipes that will tantalize your taste buds.

- **Portion Control:** Since digestion is faster after an ileostomy, smaller, more frequent meals are often recommended. We'll provide guidance on adjusting to this new routine and help you find a portion size that works for you.

- **Identifying Trigger Foods:** Certain foods may cause discomfort or gas. This book will help you identify these potential triggers and offer delicious alternative options.

Benefits You Can Savor: The Power of a Healthy Ileostomy Diet

Following a healthy ileostomy diet offers a multitude of benefits that will have you feeling fantastic:

- **Improved Digestion:** Low-fibre foods are easier for your small intestine to absorb, reducing cramping, gas, and diarrhea.

- **Reduced Risk of Dehydration:** By eating foods that are easier to absorb fluids from, you can stay adequately hydrated and feel your best.

- **Enhanced Nutrient Absorption:** A balanced ileostomy diet ensures your body gets the essential nutrients it needs to thrive.

- **Increased Energy Levels:** Proper digestion and nutrient absorption contribute to better overall energy levels.

- **Improved Quality of Life:** Managing your ileostomy through diet can give you a sense of control and empower you to enjoy a full and active life.

A Day on a Plate: Sample Ileostomy Meal Plan

Let's take a peek at what a delicious day on the ileostomy diet might look like:

- **Breakfast:** Start your day with fluffy scrambled eggs and chopped mushrooms served on a slice of white toast. A glass of milk or a cup of unsweetened applesauce on the side adds a touch of sweetness.

- **Mid-Morning Snack:** Refuel with a protein-packed snack of Greek yogurt topped with a sprinkle of your favorite berries.

- **Lunch:** Warm up with a comforting bowl of cream of chicken soup. Pair it with some crispy white rice crackers and a handful of juicy grapes for a satisfying midday meal.

- **Afternoon Snack:** Keep your energy levels up with a classic combination – banana slices dipped in a tablespoon of creamy peanut butter.

- **Dinner:** Tonight's dinner is a feast for the senses! Enjoy baked salmon with roasted asparagus and a comforting side of mashed potatoes.

- **Evening Snack:** Wind down with a simple yet satisfying snack of rice cakes topped with a slice of low-fat cheese.

Chapter 2: Ileostomy Fundamentals: Building a Strong Foundation

Understanding Your Ileostomy's Superpower

Your ileostomy is a remarkable medical marvel! It acts as a new pathway for waste to leave your body, allowing you to heal and thrive. The end of your small intestine (ileum) is diverted through the abdominal wall, creating a stoma (opening) where waste collects in a pouch you wear externally. Pretty amazing, right?

Fueling Your Body for Success: Essential Nutrients

Think of your body as a high-performance engine. After ileostomy surgery, ensuring you have the proper fuel is essential. Here are some key nutrients to focus on:

- **Protein:** This superstar nutrient helps your body heal, repair tissues, and maintain strength. Lean meats, poultry, fish, eggs, and even creamy nut butters are all excellent sources of protein.

- **Fluids:** Water is your body's best friend, especially after ileostomy surgery. Fluids help with digestion, nutrient absorption, and preventing dehydration, a common concern following surgery.

- **Vitamins and Minerals:** These micronutrients play a vital role in overall health. Aim to incorporate a variety of colorful fruits and vegetables (cooked or low-fibre options) to ensure you're getting a good mix.

Hydration: The Secret Weapon

Water is the magic ingredient for a happy and healthy ileostomy. Since your colon is no longer present to absorb fluids from waste, staying hydrated becomes even more crucial. Here's why:

- **Smooth Sailing Digestion:** Proper hydration keeps things moving smoothly through your small intestine, reducing the risk of constipation.

- **Nutrient Absorption Powerhouse:** Water helps your body absorb essential nutrients from the food you eat.

- **Electrolyte Balance for the Win:** Electrolytes are minerals that help your body function properly. Drinking enough fluids helps maintain a healthy electrolyte balance.

Protein Power: Building and Maintaining Strength

Protein is a champion for healing and overall health. Here's how it benefits you:

- **Healing Warrior:** Protein is essential for repairing tissues and rebuilding strength after surgery.

- **Energy Booster:** Feeling sluggish? Protein can help keep your energy levels up throughout the day.

- **Muscle Maintenance Marvel:** Protein helps maintain strong muscles, which is important for overall well-being.

Taming the Fibre Dragon: Why Low-Fibre is Your Friend

Dietary fibre, while essential for most people, can be a bit of a challenge for your ileostomy. Here's why:

- **Keeping Things Gentle:** High-fibre foods can be difficult for your small intestine to digest, potentially causing cramping, gas, and blockages.

- **Speedy Transit:** After surgery, food moves through your digestive system quicker. Low-fibre options are easier for your small intestine to handle and absorb nutrients from.

Stoma Care: Diet Plays a Part

Your stoma is a vital part of your digestive system, and diet can play a role in its health. Here's how:

- **Hydration Hero:** Drinking plenty of fluids helps keep your stool output soft, which can make emptying your pouch and stoma care easier.

- **Certain Foods and Output:** Be mindful of foods that may cause gas or loose stools, as this can make stoma care more frequent or messy.

Gas and Blockages: Keeping Things Moving Smoothly

Gas and blockages are occasional occurrences that some people experience with an ileostomy. Here are some tips for managing them:

- **Identify Culprits:** Keep a food diary to identify any foods that seem to trigger gas or blockages.

- **Chew Chew Chew:** Proper chewing helps break down food particles, making digestion easier.

- **Hydration is Key:** Remember, staying hydrated helps prevent constipation, which can contribute to blockages.

Chapter 3: Living Your Best Life with an Ileostomy

Food, Fun, and Freedom

An ileostomy doesn't have to hold you back from living a full and vibrant life. This chapter is your guide to navigating the world with confidence, from conquering travel adventures to mastering social gatherings.

Ileostomy and Travel: The World Awaits!

You dream of exploring new cultures, indulging in exotic cuisines, and creating unforgettable travel memories. With a little planning, your ileostomy can be your travel companion, not a limitation. Here are some tips for a smooth journey:

- **Pack Smart:** Bring along essential supplies like stoma pouches, adhesive remover wipes, and a change of clothes. Pack medications in your carry-on luggage.

- **Research is Key:** Familiarize yourself with local medical facilities in your destination, just in case. Consider packing a doctor's note explaining your ileostomy in case of language barriers.

- **Hydration Hero on the Go:** Carry a reusable water bottle and stay hydrated, especially during travel when routines might be disrupted.

- **Ileostomy-Friendly Snacks:** Pack low-fibre snacks like crackers, nut butters, and applesauce to keep you fueled throughout your adventures.

Eating Out with Confidence: Delicious Adventures Await

Restaurants don't have to be off-limits! Here's how to enjoy eating out with ease:

- **Be Prepared:** Research menus beforehand and choose low-fibre options. Don't hesitate to ask questions about ingredients.

- **Bring Back-Up:** Pack a small pouch and any necessary supplies in case you need them.

- **Communicate Clearly:** If needed, politely explain your ileostomy to your server and ask about suitable menu choices.

- **Focus on Flavor:** With a little planning, you can still enjoy delicious meals while following your ileostomy diet.

Ileostomy and Social Activities: Embrace Your Fun Side!

Social gatherings are a chance to connect with loved ones and create lasting memories. Here's how to navigate social situations with confidence:

- **Be Open:** Talk to close friends and family about your ileostomy. Understanding can go a long way in creating a comfortable and supportive environment.

- **Plan Ahead:** If you're unsure about food options at a gathering, offer to bring a dish you can enjoy.

- **Focus on the Fun:** Don't let your ileostomy limit your enjoyment. Dance the night away, participate in activities, and focus on creating happy memories.

Managing Emotional Wellbeing After Surgery

Adjusting to life with an ileostomy is a process, and it's normal to experience a range of emotions. Here are some tips for managing your emotional well-being:

- **Connect with Others:** Talk to friends, family, or a support group for ostomy patients. Sharing experiences with others who understand can be incredibly helpful.

- **Celebrate Your Achievements:** Focus on the progress you've made and the things you can still do.

- **Seek Professional Help:** If you're struggling emotionally, don't hesitate to seek professional help from a therapist or counselor.

Questions for Your Doctor

Don't be afraid to ask your doctor questions! Here are some prompts to get you started:

- What specific foods should I avoid or limit?

- Are there any vitamin or mineral supplements I should consider?

- How often should I have my stoma checked?

- What resources are available for ostomy patients?

Remember, you are not alone on this journey. With the right knowledge, planning, and a positive attitude, you can live a full and vibrant life with your ileostomy.

Part 2: Ileostomy Diet in Action – Recipes and Meal Plans

Chapter 4: Building Your Ileostomy

Pantry

A Haven for Delicious Possibilities

Imagine opening your pantry and seeing a treasure trove of ingredients ready to be transformed into delicious and nourishing ileostomy-friendly meals. This chapter equips you with the knowledge to stock your kitchen for success, navigate the grocery store with ease, and discover essential tools to become an ileostomy kitchen whiz!

Stocking Your Kitchen for Success: Must-Have Staples

Think of your pantry as a foundation for creating countless culinary masterpieces. Here are some essential ileostomy-friendly staples to get you started:

- **Low-Fibre Grains:** White bread, pasta, and rice are excellent choices for building the base of your meals. You can also explore options like cornbread or low-fibre crackers.

- **Protein Powerhouses:** Lean meats, poultry, and fish are fantastic sources of protein for healing and maintaining strength. Canned options and pre-cooked chicken breasts can be lifesavers for busy days. Eggs and nut butters are also protein-packed pantry staples.

- **Canned Goods:** Canned vegetables (drained for lower sodium content) offer a convenient and affordable way to add variety to your meals. Canned low-fibre fruits like applesauce and pears are also great options.

- **Hydration Heroes:** Stock up on bottled water to ensure you stay hydrated throughout the day. Consider flavor-infused water options for a refreshing twist.

- **Healthy Fats:** Healthy fats like olive oil, avocado oil, and nut butters provide essential nutrients and add flavor to your meals.

- **Condiment Classics:** Salt, pepper, herbs, and spices can transform simple dishes into flavorful creations. Be mindful of strong spices that may irritate your stoma.

Smart Shopping Strategies: Finding Healthy and Affordable Options

Grocery shopping doesn't have to break the bank! Here are some tips for finding healthy and affordable ileostomy-friendly ingredients:

- **Make a List, Check It Twice:** Planning your meals and creating a grocery list helps you avoid impulse purchases and stick to your budget.

- **Embrace Generic Brands:** Many generic brands offer the same quality as name brands at a lower cost.

- **Seasonal Savvy:** Seasonal fruits and vegetables are often more affordable and taste their best.

- **Sale Section Superstars:** Don't be afraid to explore the sale section for deals on protein sources and canned goods.

- **Bulk Options (if manageable):** Buying certain staples like rice or pasta in bulk can be cost-effective, but make sure you have storage space to maintain freshness.

Essential Kitchen Tools for Preparing Ileostomy-Friendly Meals

With a few key tools, your kitchen can become a haven for creating delicious and nutritious ileostomy meals. Here's what you'll need:

- **Sharp Knives:** A good chef's knife and a paring knife are essential for chopping and prepping ingredients.

- **Cutting Boards:** Use separate cutting boards for raw meat and vegetables to prevent cross-contamination.

- **Pots and Pans:** A set of pots and pans in various sizes allows you to boil, simmer, saute, and bake with ease.

- **Blender/Immersion Blender:** These tools are fantastic for creating smooth soups, purees, and protein shakes.

- **Food Storage Containers:** Leftovers are your friend! Having a variety of storage containers allows you to portion out meals and save time throughout the week.

Remember, a well-stocked pantry and a few essential tools are all you need to embark on a delicious culinary adventure with your ileostomy. The next chapter dives into a world of flavorful recipes, ready to transform your kitchen into a haven for creativity and enjoyment!

Chapter 5: Ileostomy Diet Breakfast Recipes:

Delicious Mornings Made Easy

Mornings are a chance to set the tone for a healthy and delicious day. With these ileostomy-friendly breakfast recipes, you can fuel your body with essential nutrients while enjoying a variety of flavorful options.

Remember:

- Start with small portions of new foods and see how you tolerate them.

- Drink plenty of fluids throughout the day to stay hydrated.

- Feel free to adjust portion sizes and ingredients to suit your taste preferences.

Let's get cooking!

1. Creamy Berry Protein Smoothie

This smoothie is packed with protein and low in fibre, making it a perfect way to start your day. The berries add a touch of sweetness and antioxidants.

Ingredients:

- 1 cup unsweetened almond milk (or lactose-free milk)

- 1/2 cup frozen mixed berries

- 1 scoop vanilla protein powder

- 1/4 cup plain Greek yogurt (or lactose-free yogurt)

- Handful of ice cubes (optional)

Instructions:

1. Combine all ingredients in a blender and blend until smooth and creamy.

2. Add more almond milk for a thinner consistency, or more ice cubes for a thicker smoothie.

3. Pour into a glass and enjoy!

Nutritional Information (per serving):

- Calories: 250

- Protein: 20g

- Carbohydrates: 20g

- Fat: 5g

2. Scrambled Eggs with Sauteed Spinach and Mushrooms

Eggs are a classic breakfast option, and for good reason! They're a great source of protein and can be easily customized with your favorite low-fibre ingredients.

Ingredients:

- 2 eggs

- 1 tablespoon olive oil

- 1/2 cup chopped spinach

- 1/4 cup sliced mushrooms

- Salt and pepper to taste

Instructions:

1. In a non-stick pan, heat olive oil over medium heat.

2. Add the spinach and mushrooms and cook until softened, about 2-3 minutes.

3. In a separate bowl, whisk together the eggs.

4. Pour the egg mixture into the pan with the vegetables and cook, stirring occasionally, until the eggs are set to your desired doneness.

5. Season with salt and pepper to taste.

6. Serve immediately with a slice of white toast or gluten-free bread.

Nutritional Information (per serving):

- Calories: 200

- Protein: 12g

- Carbohydrates: 7g

- Fat: 10g

3. Protein Pancakes with Berries and Low-Fat Yogurt

Pancakes don't have to be off-limits with an ileostomy diet! This recipe uses low-fibre ingredients to create fluffy and delicious pancakes you'll love.

Ingredients:

- 1/2 cup all-purpose flour

- 1 teaspoon baking powder

- 1/4 teaspoon salt

- 1 tablespoon sugar

- 1 egg

- 1/2 cup unsweetened almond milk (or lactose-free milk)

- 1 tablespoon melted butter

- 1/4 cup fresh berries (optional)

- 1/4 cup low-fat yogurt (optional)

Instructions:

1. In a medium bowl, whisk together flour, baking powder, salt, and sugar.

2. In a separate bowl, whisk together the egg, almond milk, and melted butter.

3. Pour the wet ingredients into the dry ingredients and mix until just combined. Do not overmix.

4. Heat a lightly greased non-stick pan over medium heat.

5. Pour 1/4 cup batter per pancake onto the pan.

6. If using berries, gently press a few berries into the top of each pancake.

7. Cook for 2-3 minutes per side, or until golden brown and cooked through.

8. Serve pancakes with a dollop of low-fat yogurt and additional berries (optional).

Nutritional Information (per serving without yogurt and berries):

- Calories: 200

- Protein: 5g

- Carbohydrates: 30g

- Fat: 8g

4. Baked Oatmeal with Apples and Cinnamon

Baked oatmeal is a warm and comforting breakfast option that's perfect for meal prepping. This recipe uses low-fibre ingredients and is packed with flavor.

Ingredients:

- 1/2 cup rolled oats

- 1 cup unsweetened almond milk (or lactose-free milk)

- 1/4 cup water

- 1/2 apple, peeled and diced

- 1/4 teaspoon ground cinnamon

- 1 tablespoon chopped walnuts (optional)

- 1 tablespoon honey (optional)

Instructions:

1. Preheat oven to 375°F (190°C). Lightly grease a small baking dish.

2. In a medium bowl, combine rolled oats, almond milk, water, diced apple, and cinnamon.

3. Pour the mixture into the prepared baking dish.

4. Sprinkle with chopped walnuts (optional) and drizzle with honey (optional).

5. Bake for 20-25 minutes, or until the oatmeal is set and slightly golden brown on top.

6. Let cool slightly before serving.

Nutritional Information (per serving):

- Calories: 250

- Protein: 5g

- Carbohydrates: 40g

- Fat: 5g

5. Cottage Cheese Bowl with Fruit and Granola

This breakfast bowl is a great way to get a dose of protein and calcium. You can customize it with your favorite low-fibre fruits and granola.

Ingredients:

- 1/2 cup low-fat cottage cheese

- 1/4 cup sliced strawberries

- 1/4 cup blueberries

- 1/4 cup low-fibre granola

Instructions:

1. In a bowl, combine cottage cheese, strawberries, blueberries, and granola.

2. Enjoy!

Nutritional Information (per serving):

- Calories: 200

- Protein: 15g

- Carbohydrates: 25g

- Fat: 5g

6. Egg Muffins with Sausage and Cheese

Egg muffins are a great make-ahead breakfast option. They're portable, protein-packed, and perfect for busy mornings.

Ingredients:

- 6 eggs

- 1/4 cup chopped cooked sausage (optional)

- 1/4 cup shredded cheddar cheese

- 1/4 cup chopped spinach (optional)

- Salt and pepper to taste

Instructions:

1. Preheat oven to 375°F (190°C). Grease a muffin tin.

2. In a large bowl, whisk together eggs.

3. Fold in cooked sausage, cheese, spinach (optional), salt, and pepper.

4. Pour the egg mixture into the prepared muffin tin.

5. Bake for 15-20 minutes, or until the eggs are set and cooked through.

6. Let cool slightly before serving.

Nutritional Information (per serving):

- Calories: 200

- Protein: 12g

- Carbohydrates: 5g

- Fat: 15g (with sausage)

7. Smoothie Bowl with Peanut Butter and Banana

This smoothie bowl is a fun and flavorful way to start your day. It's packed with protein, healthy fats, and potassium.

Ingredients:

- 1 cup unsweetened almond milk (or lactose-free milk)

- 1/2 banana, frozen

- 1 tablespoon peanut butter

- 1/4 cup granola

- 1/4 cup sliced banana (optional)

Instructions:

1. In a blender, combine almond milk, frozen banana, and peanut butter. Blend until smooth and creamy.

2. Pour the smoothie into a bowl.

3. Top with granola and sliced banana (optional).

Nutritional Information (per serving):

- Calories: 300

- Protein: 10g

- Carbohydrates: 40g

- Fat: 10g

8. Scrambled Tofu with Peppers and Onions

Tofu is a great plant-based source of protein. This recipe is a delicious and healthy way to start your day.

Ingredients:

- 1 block (14 oz) firm tofu, drained and pressed

- 1 tablespoon olive oil

- 1/2 green pepper, chopped

- 1/2 onion, chopped

- 1/4 teaspoon turmeric

- Salt and pepper to taste

- Chopped fresh herbs (optional)

Instructions:

1. Crumble the tofu into a bowl.

2. In a non-stick pan, heat olive oil over medium heat.

3. Add the green pepper and onion and cook until softened, about 5 minutes.

4. Add the crumbled tofu and turmeric to the pan and cook for another 5 minutes, stirring occasionally.

5. Season with salt and pepper to taste.

6. Serve immediately with chopped fresh herbs (optional) and a slice of whole-wheat toast (optional).

Nutritional Information (per serving):

- Calories: 250

- Protein: 20g

- Carbohydrates: 15g

- Fat: 15g (depending on oil used)

9. Chia Seed Pudding with Berries and Nuts

Chia seed pudding is a healthy and delicious breakfast option that's perfect for meal prepping. It's packed with fiber (but low in insoluble fiber), protein, and healthy fats. **Note:** While chia seeds are a good source of fiber, most of it is insoluble fiber, which is generally well-tolerated by people with ileostomies.

Ingredients:

- 1/4 cup chia seeds

- 1 cup unsweetened almond milk (or lactose-free milk)

- 1/4 teaspoon vanilla extract

- 1/4 cup fresh berries

- 1 tablespoon chopped nuts (optional)

Instructions:

1. In a jar or container, combine chia seeds, almond milk, and vanilla extract.

2. Stir well and refrigerate overnight, or for at least 4 hours.

3. In the morning, stir the pudding and top with fresh berries and chopped nuts (optional).

Nutritional Information (per serving):

- Calories: 250

- Protein: 5g

- Carbohydrates: 20g

- Fat: 10g

10. Low-Fibre Breakfast Burrito

This breakfast burrito is a fun and portable way to start your day. It's packed with protein and low-fibre ingredients.

Ingredients:

- 1 whole wheat tortilla (or low-fibre alternative)

- 2 scrambled eggs

- 1/4 cup diced cooked chicken breast or sausage (optional)

- 1/4 cup shredded cheese

- Salsa to taste

Instructions:

1. Warm a whole wheat tortilla (or low-fibre alternative) in a dry skillet or microwave.

2. Spread scrambled eggs onto the tortilla.

3. Top with diced chicken breast or sausage (optional), cheese, and salsa.

4. Fold the tortilla into a burrito shape and enjoy!

Nutritional Information (per serving):

- Calories: 300

- Protein: 20g (with chicken or sausage)

- Carbohydrates: 30g

- Fat: 15g (with chicken or sausage)

Chapter 6: Ileostomy Diet Lunchtime Feasts

Delicious and Filling Meals

Lunchtime is a chance to refuel and recharge for the rest of your day. With these ileostomy-friendly recipes, you can create satisfying and flavorful meals that won't compromise your dietary needs.

1. Turkey and Havarti Club Wrap

This wrap is packed with protein and low-fibre ingredients, making it a perfect lunchtime choice. The havarti cheese adds a creamy touch, while the lettuce and tomato provide a refreshing crunch.

Ingredients:

- 1 large whole wheat tortilla (or low-fibre alternative)

- 3 slices sliced turkey breast

- 1 slice havarti cheese

- 1/4 cup shredded lettuce

- 1 sliced tomato

- 1 tablespoon light mayonnaise (or low-fat yogurt)

- Mustard (optional)

Instructions:

1. Spread mayonnaise (or yogurt) on one half of the tortilla.

2. Layer turkey breast, havarti cheese, lettuce, and tomato on top of the mayonnaise (or yogurt).

3. Add mustard (optional) for a touch of spice.

4. Fold the bottom of the tortilla over the filling, then fold in the sides.

5. Roll up the tortilla tightly and enjoy!

Nutritional Information (per serving):

- Calories: 300

- Protein: 20g

- Carbohydrates: 30g

- Fat: 10g

2. Creamy Tomato Soup with Grilled Cheese

This classic comfort food duo is easily adapted for an ileostomy diet. The creamy tomato soup is smooth and easy to digest, while the grilled cheese uses low-fibre bread and cheese.

Ingredients (Soup):

- 1 tablespoon olive oil

- 1 small onion, chopped

- 1 clove garlic, minced

- 1 (14.5 oz) can diced tomatoes, undrained

- 1/2 cup chicken broth

- 1/4 cup unsweetened almond milk (or lactose-free milk)

- Salt and pepper to taste

Ingredients (Grilled Cheese):

- 2 slices white bread

- 1 slice low-fat cheddar cheese

Instructions (Soup):

1. In a saucepan, heat olive oil over medium heat.

2. Add onion and cook until softened, about 5 minutes.

3. Add garlic and cook for an additional minute.

4. Stir in diced tomatoes, chicken broth, and almond milk (or milk).

5. Bring to a simmer and cook for 10 minutes.

6. Remove from heat and blend with an immersion blender or in a blender until smooth.

7. Season with salt and pepper to taste.

Instructions (Grilled Cheese):

1. Heat a non-stick pan over medium heat.

2. Place one slice of bread in the pan.

3. Top with a slice of cheese.

4. Add the other slice of bread on top of the cheese.

5. Cook for 2-3 minutes per side, or until golden brown and cheese is melted.

Nutritional Information (per serving):

- Calories: 350

- Protein: 15g

- Carbohydrates: 40g

- Fat: 15g

3. Leftover Chicken Salad on a Bed of Greens

Leftover chicken can be transformed into a delicious and nutritious lunch. This recipe uses low-fibre ingredients and is served on a bed of greens for added vitamins and fiber.

Ingredients:

- 1 cup chopped cooked chicken breast

- 1/4 cup chopped celery

- 1 tablespoon light mayonnaise (or low-fat yogurt)

- Salt and pepper to taste

- Mixed greens (choose low-fibre varieties like romaine or iceberg lettuce)

Instructions:

1. In a bowl, combine chopped chicken breast, celery, mayonnaise (or yogurt), salt, and pepper.

2. Toss to coat.

3. Place a bed of mixed greens on a plate.

4. Top with the chicken salad mixture and enjoy!

Nutritional Information (per serving):

- Calories: 250

- Protein: 25g

- Carbohydrates: 5g

- Fat: 10g

4. Tuna Salad Sandwich with Wheat Sprouts

This light and refreshing sandwich is perfect for a hot summer day. Tuna salad is a great source of protein, and wheat sprouts add a touch of vitamins and a pleasant crunch.

Ingredients:

- 2 slices white bread

- 1 can (5 oz) canned tuna in water, drained

- 1 tablespoon light mayonnaise (or low-fat yogurt)

- 1 tablespoon chopped celery

- Salt and pepper to taste

- 1/4 cup alfalfa sprouts (or other low-fibre sprouts)

Instructions:

1. In a bowl, combine tuna, mayonnaise (or yogurt), celery, salt, and pepper.

2. Spread the tuna salad mixture onto one slice of bread.

3. Top with alfalfa sprouts (or other low-fibre sprouts).

4. Add the other slice of bread on top and enjoy!

Nutritional Information (per serving):

- Calories: 300

- Protein: 20g

- Carbohydrates: 35g

- Fat: 5g

5. Creamy Avocado Pasta Salad

This pasta salad is a flavorful and satisfying lunch option. Creamy avocado adds richness, while cherry tomatoes and peas provide a burst of color and freshness.

Ingredients:

- 1 cup cooked pasta (such as penne or rotini)
- 1/2 avocado, mashed
- 1/4 cup cherry tomatoes, halved
- 1/4 cup cooked peas
- 1 tablespoon lemon juice
- Salt and pepper to taste

Instructions:

1. In a large bowl, combine cooked pasta, mashed avocado, cherry tomatoes, peas, lemon juice, salt, and pepper.
2. Toss to coat and enjoy!

Nutritional Information (per serving):

- Calories: 350

- Protein: 5g

- Carbohydrates: 40g

- Fat: 15g

6. Leftover Salmon with Roasted Vegetables

Roasted vegetables are a healthy and delicious way to add variety to your lunch routine. This recipe uses leftover salmon for a protein boost.

Ingredients:

- 4 oz leftover baked salmon

- 1 cup chopped broccoli florets

- 1/2 cup chopped carrots

- 1 tablespoon olive oil

- Salt and pepper to taste

Instructions:

1. Preheat oven to 400°F (200°C).

2. Toss broccoli and carrots with olive oil, salt, and pepper.

3. Spread vegetables on a baking sheet and roast for 20-25 minutes, or until tender-crisp.

4. Flake the leftover salmon.

5. Serve roasted vegetables with flaked salmon and enjoy!

Nutritional Information (per serving):

- Calories: 300

- Protein: 25g

- Carbohydrates: 20g

- Fat: 15g

7. Chicken Caesar Salad

This classic salad is easily adapted for an ileostomy diet. Use low-fibre romaine lettuce and a light Caesar dressing for a delicious and satisfying lunch.

Ingredients:

- 2 cups chopped romaine lettuce

- 4 oz grilled or baked chicken breast, sliced

- 1/4 cup shredded Parmesan cheese

- 2 tablespoons light Caesar dressing

- Croutons (optional, choose low-fibre options)

Instructions:

1. In a large bowl, combine romaine lettuce, chicken breast, Parmesan cheese, and Caesar dressing.

2. Toss to coat.

3. Top with croutons (optional) and enjoy!

Nutritional Information (per serving):

- Calories: 350

- Protein: 30g

- Carbohydrates: 5g

- Fat: 15g (with croutons)

8. Egg Salad Lettuce Wraps

Egg salad is a versatile and protein-packed lunch option. This recipe uses lettuce wraps instead of bread for a low-fibre alternative.

Ingredients:

- 2 hard-boiled eggs, chopped

- 1 tablespoon light mayonnaise (or low-fat yogurt)

- 1 tablespoon chopped celery

- 1/4 teaspoon dried dill

- Salt and pepper to taste

- 4 large lettuce leaves (such as romaine or butter lettuce)

Instructions:

1. In a bowl, combine chopped eggs, mayonnaise (or yogurt), celery, dill, salt, and pepper.

2. Wash and dry lettuce leaves.

3. Place a scoop of egg salad in each lettuce leaf and enjoy!

Nutritional Information (per serving):

- Calories: 200

- Protein: 12g

- Carbohydrates: 5g

- Fat: 10g

9. Turkey and Vegetable Skewers with Hummus

This recipe is a fun and interactive way to enjoy lunch. Lean turkey and colorful vegetables are grilled on skewers and served with a creamy hummus dip.

Ingredients:

- 1 cup cubed cooked turkey breast

- 1/2 cup cherry tomatoes

- 1/2 cup zucchini, cut into chunks

- 1/2 cup red bell pepper, cut into chunks

- 1 tablespoon olive oil

- Salt and pepper to taste

- 1/2 cup hummus

Instructions:

1. Preheat grill or grill pan to medium heat.

2. Thread cubed turkey breast, cherry tomatoes, zucchini chunks, and red bell pepper chunks onto skewers.

3. Brush with olive oil and season with salt and pepper.

4. Grill for 5-7 minutes per side, or until cooked through.

5. Serve skewers with hummus for dipping and enjoy!

Nutritional Information (per serving):

- Calories: 350

- Protein: 25g

- Carbohydrates: 20g

- Fat: 15g

10. Creamy Cottage Cheese Fruit Bowl

This refreshing and healthy dessert can also be a satisfying light lunch option. Cottage cheese provides protein and calcium, while fruit adds sweetness and vitamins.

Ingredients:

- 1/2 cup low-fat cottage cheese
- 1/2 cup sliced strawberries
- 1/4 cup blueberries
- 1 tablespoon honey (optional)

Instructions:

1. In a bowl, combine cottage cheese, strawberries, and blueberries.
2. Drizzle with honey (optional) and enjoy!

Nutritional Information (per serving):

- Calories: 200

- Protein: 15g

- Carbohydrates: 20g

- Fat: 5g

These are just a few ideas to get you started on your ileostomy lunch adventure. With a little creativity, you can create delicious and nutritious meals that fit your dietary needs. Remember to listen to your body and adjust portion sizes and ingredients as needed. Enjoy!

Chapter 6: Ileostomy Diet Dinnertime Dreams

Delicious and Satisfying Meals

Dinnertime is a chance to unwind, connect with loved ones, and enjoy a delicious and nourishing meal. With an ileostomy, you can still create flavorful and satisfying dishes that meet your dietary needs.

1. Baked Lemon Chicken with Roasted Asparagus

This classic dish is simple to prepare and perfect for a weeknight meal. The lemon adds a bright flavor to the chicken, while the roasted asparagus provides a dose of vitamins.

Ingredients:

- 4 boneless, skinless chicken breasts

- 2 tablespoons olive oil

- 1 tablespoon lemon juice

- 1 teaspoon dried oregano

- 1/2 teaspoon garlic powder

- Salt and pepper to taste

- 1 pound asparagus, trimmed

Instructions:

1. Preheat oven to 400°F (200°C).

2. In a bowl, whisk together olive oil, lemon juice, oregano, garlic powder, salt, and pepper.

3. Place chicken breasts in a baking dish and pour the marinade over them.

4. Toss to coat.

5. Arrange asparagus spears around the chicken breasts.

6. Bake for 25-30 minutes, or until chicken is cooked through and asparagus is tender-crisp.

Nutritional Information (per serving):

- Calories: 300

- Protein: 30g

- Carbohydrates: 15g

- Fat: 15g

2. Salmon with Creamy Dill Sauce and Rice

Salmon is a great source of omega-3 fatty acids, which are beneficial for heart health. This recipe features a creamy dill sauce that complements the flavor of the fish perfectly.

Ingredients:

- 4 salmon fillets

- 1 tablespoon olive oil

- 1/2 cup low-fat milk (or lactose-free milk)

- 1/4 cup light cream cheese

- 1 tablespoon chopped fresh dill (or 1 teaspoon dried dill)

- Salt and pepper to taste

- 1 cup cooked white rice

Instructions:

1. Heat olive oil in a skillet over medium heat.

2. Season salmon fillets with salt and pepper.

3. Add salmon to the skillet and cook for 4-5 minutes per side, or until cooked through.

4. In a separate saucepan, whisk together milk, cream cheese, dill, salt, and pepper.

5. Heat over medium heat until the sauce is smooth and thickened.

6. Serve salmon over cooked rice and spoon the creamy dill sauce over the top.

Nutritional Information (per serving):

- Calories: 400

- Protein: 30g

- Carbohydrates: 30g

- Fat: 15g

3. One-Pot Creamy Tomato Pasta with Chicken Sausage

This one-pot pasta dish is a lifesaver on busy weeknights. It's packed with protein and flavor, and only requires one pot for easy cleanup.

Ingredients:

- 1 tablespoon olive oil

- 1 pound boneless, skinless chicken sausage, sliced

- 1 onion, chopped

- 2 cloves garlic, minced

- 1 (14.5 oz) can diced tomatoes, undrained

- 1/2 cup chicken broth

- 1/4 cup heavy cream (or lactose-free heavy cream)

- 1/4 cup grated Parmesan cheese

- 1 cup penne pasta

- Salt and pepper to taste

Instructions:

1. Heat olive oil in a large pot or Dutch oven over medium heat.

2. Add chicken sausage and cook until browned.

3. Add onion and garlic and cook until softened, about 5 minutes.

4. Stir in diced tomatoes, chicken broth, heavy cream, Parmesan cheese, and penne pasta.

5. Bring to a boil, then reduce heat and simmer for 10-12 minutes, or until pasta is cooked through and sauce has thickened.

6. Season with salt and pepper to taste.

Nutritional Information (per serving):

- Calories: 450

- Protein: 25g

- Carbohydrates: 40g

- Fat: 20g

4. Turkey Shepherd's Pie

This comforting dish is a hearty and satisfying meal. Ground turkey replaces traditional ground lamb, making it a lower-fat option. Mashed potatoes provide a creamy topping.

Ingredients:

- 1 tablespoon olive oil

- 1 pound ground turkey

- 1 onion, chopped

- 2 carrots, chopped

- 1 celery stalk, chopped

- 1 cup frozen peas

- 1 (14.5 oz) can diced tomatoes, undrained

- 1/2 cup beef broth

- 1 tablespoon Worcestershire sauce

- 1 teaspoon dried thyme

- Salt and pepper to taste

- 4 cups peeled and mashed potatoes (made with low-fat milk or lactose-free milk)

Instructions:

1. Preheat oven to 400°F (200°C).

2. Heat olive oil in a large skillet over medium heat.

3. Add ground turkey and cook until browned, breaking it up with a spoon.

4. Drain any excess fat.

5. Add onion, carrots, and celery to the skillet and cook until softened, about 5 minutes.

6. Stir in frozen peas, diced tomatoes, beef broth, Worcestershire sauce, and thyme.

7. Season with salt and pepper to taste.

8. Bring to a simmer and cook for 5 minutes.

9. Transfer the meat mixture to a baking dish.

10. Top with mashed potatoes, spreading evenly to cover the meat mixture.

11. Bake for 20-25 minutes, or until the potatoes are golden brown and the filling is bubbly.

Nutritional Information (per serving):

- Calories: 450

- Protein: 35g

- Carbohydrates: 40g

- Fat: 20g

5. Beef and Vegetable Stir-Fry with Rice Noodles

This stir-fry is a quick and easy way to get your protein and vegetable fix. Lean beef and colorful vegetables are stir-fried together for a flavorful and satisfying meal.

Ingredients:

- 1 tablespoon olive oil

- 1 pound flank steak, sliced thinly

- 1 red bell pepper, sliced

- 1 green bell pepper, sliced

- 1 cup broccoli florets

- 1/2 cup snow peas

- 1/4 cup low-sodium soy sauce

- 1 tablespoon cornstarch

- 1 tablespoon rice vinegar

- 1 teaspoon grated ginger

- 1/2 teaspoon sesame oil

- 8 oz rice noodles, cooked according to package directions

Instructions:

1. In a small bowl, whisk together soy sauce, cornstarch, rice vinegar, ginger, and sesame oil.

2. Heat olive oil in a large skillet or wok over high heat.

3. Add beef and cook for 2-3 minutes, or until browned.

4. Add bell peppers, broccoli florets, and snow peas to the skillet and cook for an additional 3-4 minutes, or until vegetables are tender-crisp.

5. Pour the soy sauce mixture into the skillet and bring to a simmer.

6. Cook for 1 minute, or until the sauce thickens slightly.

7. Serve over cooked rice noodles.

Nutritional Information (per serving):

- Calories: 400

- Protein: 30g

- Carbohydrates: 40g

- Fat: 15g

6. Baked Cod with Lemon Herb Butter and Roasted Brussels Sprouts

This recipe is a light and flavorful option for a healthy dinner. The lemon herb butter adds a touch of brightness to the cod, while the roasted Brussels sprouts provide a satisfying side dish.

Ingredients:

- 4 cod fillets

- 2 tablespoons olive oil

- 1 tablespoon lemon juice

- 1/2 teaspoon dried parsley

- 1/4 teaspoon dried thyme

- 1/4 cup unsalted butter, softened

- Salt and pepper to taste

- 1 pound Brussels sprouts, trimmed and halved

Instructions:

1. Preheat oven to 400°F (200°C).

2. In a bowl, whisk together olive oil, lemon juice, parsley, and thyme.

3. Brush the cod fillets with the olive oil mixture.

4. Season with salt and pepper.

5. In a separate bowl, mash together the softened butter with additional chopped parsley (optional).

6. Place cod fillets on a baking sheet.

7. Top each fillet with a pat of lemon herb butter.

8. Toss Brussels sprouts with olive oil, salt, and pepper.

9. Arrange the Brussels sprouts around the cod fillets on the baking sheet.

10. Bake for 15-20 minutes, or until the cod is cooked through and flaky and the Brussels sprouts are tender-crisp.

Nutritional Information (per serving):

- Calories: 400

- Protein: 35g

- Carbohydrates: 20g

- Fat: 20g

7. Creamy Chicken Noodle Soup

This classic comfort food is perfect for a chilly night. This recipe uses low-fat milk and cream cheese to create a creamy soup base without compromising your ileostomy diet.

Ingredients:

- 1 tablespoon olive oil

- 1 onion, chopped

- 2 carrots, chopped

- 2 celery stalks, chopped

- 4 cups chicken broth

- 1 boneless, skinless chicken breast, cooked and shredded

- 1/2 cup low-fat milk (or lactose-free milk)

- 1/4 cup light cream cheese, softened

- 1/2 cup egg noodles

- 1/4 cup chopped fresh parsley (optional)

- Salt and pepper to taste

Instructions:

1. Heat olive oil in a large pot or Dutch oven over medium heat.

2. Add onion, carrots, and celery and cook until softened, about 5 minutes.

3. Pour in chicken broth and bring to a boil.

4. Reduce heat and simmer for 10 minutes.

5. Add shredded chicken, milk, and cream cheese to the pot.

6. Stir until the cream cheese is melted and the soup is smooth.

7. Add egg noodles and cook for an additional 5 minutes, or until the noodles are cooked through.

8. Season with salt and pepper to taste.

9. Garnish with chopped parsley (optional) and serve.

Nutritional Information (per serving):

- Calories: 350

- Protein: 30g

- Carbohydrates: 35g

- Fat: 15g

8. Baked Tilapia with Mango Salsa

This dish is a flavorful and healthy twist on traditional fish tacos. Baked tilapia is topped with a refreshing mango salsa for a burst of sweetness and acidity.

Ingredients:

- 4 tilapia fillets

- 2 tablespoons olive oil

- 1/2 teaspoon chili powder

- 1/4 teaspoon cumin

- Salt and pepper to taste

- 1 ripe mango, diced

- 1/2 red bell pepper, diced

- 1/4 red onion, diced

- 1 tablespoon lime juice

- 1/4 cup chopped fresh cilantro

Instructions:

1. Preheat oven to 400°F (200°C).

2. In a bowl, toss tilapia fillets with olive oil, chili powder, cumin, salt, and pepper.

3. Arrange the tilapia fillets on a baking sheet.

4. In a separate bowl, combine diced mango, red bell pepper, red onion, lime juice, and chopped cilantro.

5. Spoon the mango salsa over the top of the tilapia fillets.

6. Bake for 15-20 minutes, or until the tilapia is cooked through and flaky.

Nutritional Information (per serving):

- Calories: 350

- Protein: 30g

- Carbohydrates: 30g

- Fat: 10g

9. Lentil and Vegetable Curry

This hearty lentil curry is a vegetarian option packed with protein and fiber. It's a flavorful and satisfying meal that's perfect for a cold night.

Ingredients:

- 1 tablespoon olive oil

- 1 onion, chopped

- 2 cloves garlic, minced

- 1 teaspoon curry powder

- 1/2 teaspoon ground cumin

- 1 (14.5 oz) can diced tomatoes, undrained

- 1 cup vegetable broth

- 1 cup green lentils, rinsed

- 1 cup chopped carrots

- 1 cup chopped broccoli florets

- 1/2 cup chopped green beans

- 1 cup cooked white rice (optional)

- Salt and pepper to taste

Instructions:

1. Heat olive oil in a large pot or Dutch oven over medium heat.

2. Add onion and garlic and cook until softened, about 5 minutes.

3. Stir in curry powder and cumin and cook for an additional minute.

4. Add diced tomatoes, vegetable broth, lentils, carrots, broccoli, and green beans.

5. Bring to a boil, then reduce heat and simmer for 20-25 minutes, or until the lentils are tender.

6. Season with salt and pepper to taste.

7. Serve over cooked white rice (optional) and enjoy!

Nutritional Information (per serving):

- Calories: 400

- Protein: 18g (without rice) 25g (with rice)

- Carbohydrates: 50g (with rice) 30g (without rice)

- Fat: 15g

10. Turkey Meatballs with Marinara Sauce and Zucchini Noodles

This recipe is a fun and healthy twist on classic spaghetti and meatballs. Lean ground turkey is used for the meatballs, and zucchini noodles replace traditional spaghetti for a lower-carb option.

Ingredients:

- 1 pound ground turkey

- 1/2 cup breadcrumbs

- 1/4 cup grated Parmesan cheese

- 1 egg, beaten

- 1/4 cup chopped onion

- 1 teaspoon dried oregano

- 1/2 teaspoon garlic powder

- Salt and pepper to taste

- 1 jar (24 oz) marinara sauce

- 2 large zucchinis, spiralized

Instructions:

1. In a large bowl, combine ground turkey, breadcrumbs, Parmesan cheese, egg, onion, oregano, garlic powder, salt, and pepper.

2. Mix well and form into small meatballs.

3. Heat a large skillet over medium heat with a light coating of olive oil (optional).

4. Add meatballs to the skillet and cook for 5-7 minutes per side, or until browned on all sides.

5. Pour marinara sauce into the skillet and bring to a simmer.

6. Reduce heat and simmer for 10 minutes, or until the meatballs are cooked through and the sauce is heated through.

7. While the meatballs are simmering, spiralize the zucchinis using a spiralizer or julienne peeler.

8. Heat a separate pan with a light coating of olive oil (optional) over medium heat.

9. Add the zucchini noodles and cook for 2-3 minutes, or until tender-crisp.

10. Serve the meatballs and marinara sauce over the zucchini noodles and enjoy!

Nutritional Information (per serving):

- Calories: 400

- Protein: 30g

- Carbohydrates: 30g

- Fat: 15g

These are just a few ideas to get you started on your ileostomy dinnertime adventure. With a little creativity, you can create delicious and nutritious meals that fit your dietary needs. Remember to listen to your body and adjust portion sizes and ingredients as needed. Enjoy!

Chapter 7: Side Dishes that Shine

Having an ileostomy doesn't mean sacrificing flavor or variety when it comes to side dishes. Here are 10 delicious and ileostomy-friendly recipes that will complement any main course:

1. Creamy Mashed Potatoes

This classic comfort food is easily adapted for an ileostomy diet. Opt for low-fat milk or lactose-free milk for a creamy texture without compromising your dietary needs.

Ingredients:

- 4 medium potatoes, peeled and cubed

- 1/2 cup low-fat milk (or lactose-free milk)

- 2 tablespoons unsalted butter

- Salt and pepper to taste

Instructions:

1. In a large pot, cover potatoes with water and bring to a boil.

2. Reduce heat and simmer for 15-20 minutes, or until potatoes are tender.

3. Drain the water and return the potatoes to the pot.

4. Using a potato masher or hand mixer, mash the potatoes until smooth.

5. Gradually add milk and butter while mashing until desired consistency is reached.

6. Season with salt and pepper to taste.

Nutritional Information (per serving):

- Calories: 200

- Protein: 5g

- Carbohydrates: 35g

- Fat: 5g

2. Roasted Asparagus with Parmesan Cheese

Simple yet flavorful, roasted asparagus is a perfect low-fibre side dish. A sprinkle of Parmesan cheese adds a touch of salty richness.

Ingredients:

- 1 pound asparagus, trimmed

- 1 tablespoon olive oil

- Salt and pepper to taste

- 1/4 cup grated Parmesan cheese

Instructions:

1. Preheat oven to 400°F (200°C).

2. Toss asparagus spears with olive oil, salt, and pepper.

3. Spread asparagus on a baking sheet in a single layer.

4. Roast for 10-12 minutes, or until tender-crisp.

5. Remove from oven and sprinkle with Parmesan cheese.

Nutritional Information (per serving):

- Calories: 100

- Protein: 2g

- Carbohydrates: 15g

- Fat: 5g

3. Sautéed Green Beans with Garlic

Sauteed green beans are a quick and easy side dish that's packed with nutrients. Garlic adds a touch of savory flavor.

Ingredients:

- 1 pound green beans, trimmed and cut into bite-sized pieces

- 1 tablespoon olive oil

- 2 cloves garlic, minced

- Salt and pepper to taste

Instructions:

1. Heat olive oil in a large skillet over medium heat.

2. Add garlic and cook for 30 seconds, or until fragrant.

3. Add green beans and cook for 5-7 minutes, or until tender-crisp.

4. Season with salt and pepper to taste.

Nutritional Information (per serving):

- Calories: 75

- Protein: 2g

- Carbohydrates: 10g

- Fat: 4g

4. Creamy Butternut Squash Soup

This smooth and creamy soup is packed with flavor and low in fibre. Butternut squash provides natural sweetness, while low-fat milk creates a creamy texture.

Ingredients:

- 1 medium butternut squash, peeled and diced

- 1 onion, chopped

- 2 cloves garlic, minced

- 1 tablespoon olive oil

- 4 cups chicken broth (or vegetable broth)

- 1 cup low-fat milk (or lactose-free milk)

- Salt and pepper to taste

Instructions:

1. Heat olive oil in a large pot or Dutch oven over medium heat.

2. Add onion and garlic and cook until softened, about 5 minutes.

3. Add diced butternut squash and cook for an additional 5 minutes.

4. Pour in chicken broth and bring to a boil.

5. Reduce heat and simmer for 20-25 minutes, or until butternut squash is tender.

6. Let the soup cool slightly.

7. Using a hand blender or immersion blender, puree the soup until smooth.

8. Stir in milk and heat through.

9. Season with salt and pepper to taste.

Nutritional Information (per serving):

- Calories: 250

- Protein: 5g

- Carbohydrates: 30g

- Fat: 10g

5. Simple Herb Vinaigrette

This versatile dressing is perfect for salads, roasted vegetables, or grilled chicken. It's low in fat and packs a punch of flavor.

Ingredients:

- 1/4 cup olive oil

- 2 tablespoons lemon juice

- 1 tablespoon red wine vinegar

- 1 teaspoon Dijon mustard

- 1/2 teaspoon dried oregano

- 1/4 teaspoon dried thyme

- Salt and pepper to taste

Instructions:

1. In a small bowl, whisk together olive oil, lemon juice, red wine vinegar, Dijon mustard, oregano, thyme, salt, and pepper.

2. Store in an airtight container in the refrigerator for up to a week.

Nutritional Information (per serving):

- Calories: 100

- Protein: 0g

- Carbohydrates: 1g

- Fat: 11g

6. Creamy Cucumber Yogurt Dill Dip

This refreshing dip is perfect for crudités or crackers. Greek yogurt provides a creamy base without the high lactose content of traditional sour cream.

Ingredients:

- 1 cup plain Greek yogurt

- 1/2 medium cucumber, peeled and seeded, diced

- 1 tablespoon chopped fresh dill

- 1 tablespoon lemon juice

- Salt and pepper to taste

Instructions:

1. In a bowl, combine Greek yogurt, diced cucumber, dill, lemon juice, salt, and pepper.

2. Stir well to combine.

3. Serve chilled with your favorite vegetables or crackers.

Nutritional Information (per serving):

- Calories: 80

- Protein: 8g

- Carbohydrates: 8g

- Fat: 2g

7. Sauteed Mushrooms with Thyme

Earthy mushrooms are a delicious and low-fibre side dish. A sprinkle of thyme adds a touch of aromatic flavor.

Ingredients:

- 1 pound mushrooms, sliced

- 1 tablespoon olive oil

- 2 cloves garlic, minced

- 1/2 teaspoon dried thyme

- Salt and pepper to taste

Instructions:

1. Heat olive oil in a large skillet over medium heat.

2. Add mushrooms and cook for 5-7 minutes, or until softened and browned.

3. Add garlic and thyme and cook for an additional minute, or until fragrant.

4. Season with salt and pepper to taste.

Nutritional Information (per serving):

- Calories: 75

- Protein: 2g

- Carbohydrates: 5g

- Fat: 4g

8. Baked Sweet Potato Fries

Sweet potato fries are a healthier alternative to traditional french fries. They're naturally low in fibre and perfect for dipping in your favorite sauce.

Ingredients:

- 2 large sweet potatoes, peeled and cut into wedges

- 1 tablespoon olive oil

- Salt and pepper to taste

Instructions:

1. Preheat oven to 400°F (200°C).

2. Toss sweet potato wedges with olive oil, salt, and pepper.

3. Spread the wedges on a baking sheet in a single layer.

4. Bake for 20-25 minutes, or until golden brown and tender-crisp.

5. Flip the fries halfway through baking for even browning.

Nutritional Information (per serving):

- Calories: 200

- Protein: 1g

- Carbohydrates: 25g

- Fat: 5g

9. Lemon Herb Couscous

This light and flavorful side dish is perfect for a warm summer evening. Couscous cooks quickly and absorbs the lemon and herb flavors beautifully.

Ingredients:

- 1 cup couscous

- 1 cup chicken broth (or vegetable broth)

- 1 tablespoon olive oil

- 1 tablespoon lemon juice

- 1/4 teaspoon dried parsley

- 1/4 teaspoon dried thyme

- Salt and pepper to taste

Instructions:

1. In a saucepan, bring chicken broth to a boil.

2. Stir in couscous and remove from heat.

3. Cover the pot and let stand for 5 minutes, or until couscous is fluffy.

4. Fluff the couscous with a fork and drizzle with olive oil.

5. Stir in lemon juice, parsley, thyme, salt, and pepper.

Nutritional Information (per serving):

- Calories: 175

- Protein: 5g

- Carbohydrates: 30g

- Fat: 5g

10. Roasted Cherry Tomatoes with Balsamic Glaze

Sweet and tangy, roasted cherry tomatoes are a simple yet elegant side dish. A drizzle of balsamic glaze adds a touch of sophistication.

Ingredients:

- 1 pint cherry tomatoes

- 1 tablespoon olive oil

- Salt and pepper to taste

- 1/4 cup balsamic vinegar

- 1 tablespoon brown sugar

Instructions:

1. Preheat oven to 400°F (200°C).

2. Toss cherry tomatoes with olive oil, salt, and pepper.

3. Spread the tomatoes on a baking sheet in a single layer.

4. Roast for 20-25 minutes, or until the tomatoes are blistered and starting to burst.

5. While the tomatoes are roasting, in a small saucepan, combine balsamic vinegar and brown sugar.

6. Heat over medium heat until the mixture thickens and reduces by half, about 5-7 minutes.

7. Drizzle the balsamic glaze over the roasted cherry tomatoes before serving.

Nutritional Information (per serving):

- Calories: 75

- Protein: 1g

- Carbohydrates: 15g

- Fat: 4g

Living with an ileostomy doesn't mean you have to give up on sweet treats! Here are 10 delicious and ileostomy-friendly recipes that will satisfy your cravings without compromising your dietary needs:

1. Baked Apples with Cinnamon

This classic dessert is simple, healthy, and easily digestible. Baked apples are naturally sweet, and cinnamon adds a warm and cozy flavor.

Ingredients:

- 2 apples (such as Gala or Golden Delicious)

- 1/4 cup water

- 1 tablespoon ground cinnamon

- 1 tablespoon low-fat butter or lactose-free butter, softened (optional)

Instructions:

1. Preheat oven to 375°F (190°C).

2. Core the apples, leaving the bottom intact.

3. Place the apples in a baking dish and add water to the bottom of the dish.

4. Sprinkle the apples with cinnamon.

5. Dot with butter (optional) for added richness.

6. Bake for 30-35 minutes, or until the apples are tender and cooked through.

Nutritional Information (per serving):

- Calories: 100

- Protein: 0g

- Carbohydrates: 25g

- Fat: 5g (with butter)

2. Low-Fibre Blueberry Muffins

These muffins are moist, flavorful, and perfect for a quick breakfast or snack. Using white flour and omitting high-fibre fruits keeps them ileostomy-friendly.

Ingredients:

- 1 1/2 cups all-purpose flour

- 1/2 cup sugar

- 2 teaspoons baking powder

- 1/4 teaspoon salt

- 1 cup low-fat milk (or lactose-free milk)

- 1 egg

- 1/4 cup melted butter or canola oil

- 1 cup blueberries (fresh or frozen)

Instructions:

1. Preheat oven to 400°F (200°C).

2. In a large bowl, whisk together flour, sugar, baking powder, and salt.

3. In a separate bowl, whisk together milk, egg, and melted butter (or oil).

4. Add the wet ingredients to the dry ingredients and stir until just combined.

5. Gently fold in blueberries.

6. Fill muffin tins lined with paper liners.

7. Bake for 15-20 minutes, or until a toothpick inserted into the center comes out clean.

Nutritional Information (per serving):

- Calories: 250

- Protein: 4g

- Carbohydrates: 35g

- Fat: 10g

3. Creamy Rice Pudding with Berries

This comforting dessert is made with cooked rice, milk, and a touch of sugar for a creamy and satisfying treat.

Ingredients:

- 1 cup cooked white rice

- 1 cup low-fat milk (or lactose-free milk)

- 1/4 cup water

- 2 tablespoons sugar

- 1/2 teaspoon vanilla extract

- 1/4 cup mixed berries (such as strawberries, blueberries, raspberries)

Instructions:

1. In a saucepan, combine cooked rice, milk, water, sugar, and vanilla extract.

2. Heat over medium heat, stirring constantly, until the mixture thickens and becomes creamy, about 5-7 minutes.

3. Remove from heat and let cool slightly.

4. Spoon the pudding into bowls and top with fresh berries.

Nutritional Information (per serving):

- Calories: 200

- Protein: 4g

- Carbohydrates: 35g

- Fat: 2g

4. Yogurt Parfait with Granola and Fruit

This layered treat is packed with protein and flavor. Choose low-fibre granola and lactose-free yogurt for an ileostomy-friendly option.

Ingredients:

- 1 cup plain Greek yogurt (or lactose-free yogurt)

- 1/4 cup low-fibre granola

- 1/2 cup sliced fruit (such as strawberries, bananas, or peaches)

Instructions:

1. In a small glass or parfait dish, layer 1/3 cup of yogurt, 1/4 cup of granola, and 1/4 cup of sliced fruit.

2. Repeat the layers one more time.

3. Enjoy chilled.

Nutritional Information (per serving):

- Calories: 250

- Protein: 15g

- Carbohydrates: 30g

- Fat: 5g

5. Pumpkin Spice Smoothie

This creamy smoothie is perfect for a fall-inspired treat. Pumpkin puree adds a touch of sweetness and seasonal flavor, while low-fat milk keeps it ileostomy-friendly.

Ingredients:

- 1 cup low-fat milk (or lactose-free milk)
- 1/2 cup canned pumpkin puree
- 1/2 banana, frozen
- 1/4 teaspoon ground cinnamon
- 1/8 teaspoon ground nutmeg
- 1/4 teaspoon ground ginger
- Ice cubes (optional)

Instructions:

1. Blend all ingredients together in a blender until smooth and creamy.

2. Add ice cubes for a thicker consistency (optional).

3. Serve immediately.

Nutritional Information (per serving):

- Calories: 200

- Protein: 5g

- Carbohydrates: 30g

- Fat: 5g

6. Baked Pears with Ginger and Honey

This elegant dessert is simple to prepare and perfect for a special occasion. Baked pears are naturally sweet, and ginger and honey add a touch of warmth and complexity.

Ingredients:

- 2 ripe pears

- 1 tablespoon honey

- 1/2 teaspoon grated ginger

- 1/4 teaspoon ground cinnamon

- 1 tablespoon water

Instructions:

1. Preheat oven to 375°F (190°C).

2. Core the pears, leaving the bottom intact.

3. Place the pears in a baking dish and add water to the bottom of the dish.

4. In a small bowl, combine honey, ginger, and cinnamon.

5. Brush the pears with the honey mixture.

6. Bake for 30-35 minutes, or until the pears are tender and cooked through.

Nutritional Information (per serving):

- Calories: 200

- Protein: 0g

- Carbohydrates: 50g

- Fat: 0g

7. No-Bake Energy Bites with Dates and Nuts

These no-bake bites are a healthy and satisfying snack option. Dates provide natural sweetness, while nuts add protein and healthy fats.

Ingredients:

- 1 cup pitted dates, chopped

- 1/2 cup rolled oats

- 1/4 cup chopped nuts (such as almonds, walnuts, or pecans)

- 1 tablespoon ground cinnamon

- 1 tablespoon chia seeds (optional)

Instructions:

1. In a food processor, pulse together dates, rolled oats, nuts, cinnamon, and chia seeds (optional) until a sticky mixture forms.

2. Roll the mixture into bite-sized balls.

3. Store in an airtight container in the refrigerator for up to a week.

Nutritional Information (per serving):

- Calories: 200

- Protein: 4g

- Carbohydrates: 30g

- Fat: 10g

8. Low-Fibre Banana Bread

This moist and flavorful banana bread is perfect for breakfast or a snack. Using white flour and omitting high-fibre ingredients keeps it ileostomy-friendly.

Ingredients:

- 1 1/2 cups all-purpose flour

- 3/4 cup sugar

- 2 teaspoons baking powder

- 1/2 teaspoon salt

- 1/2 cup melted butter or canola oil

- 2 ripe bananas, mashed

- 1 egg

- 1/4 cup low-fat milk (or lactose-free milk)

- 1 teaspoon vanilla extract

Instructions:

1. Preheat oven to 350°F (175°C).

2. Grease a loaf pan.

3. In a large bowl, whisk together flour, sugar, baking powder, and salt.

4. In a separate bowl, whisk together melted butter (or oil), mashed bananas, egg, milk, and vanilla extract.

5. Pour the wet ingredients into the dry ingredients and stir until just combined.

6. Do not overmix.

7. Pour batter into the prepared loaf pan.

8. Bake for 50-60 minutes, or until a toothpick inserted into the center comes out clean.

9. Let cool in the pan for 10 minutes before transferring to a wire rack to cool completely.

Nutritional Information (per serving):

- Calories: 300

- Protein: 4g

- Carbohydrates: 40g

- Fat: 10g

9. Rice Cake Snacks with Nut Butter and Fruit

Rice cakes are a versatile base for a quick and easy sweet treat. Choose low-fibre options like nut butter and sliced fruit for an ileostomy-friendly snack.

Ingredients:

- 2 rice cakes

- 2 tablespoons nut butter (such as creamy peanut butter or almond butter)

- 1/4 cup sliced banana or strawberries

Instructions:

1. Spread nut butter on each rice cake.

2. Top with sliced banana or strawberries.

3. Enjoy!

Nutritional Information (per serving):

- Calories: 200

- Protein: 5g

- Carbohydrates: 30g

- Fat: 10g

10. Creamy Avocado Popsicles

These frozen treats are a healthy and refreshing way to satisfy your sweet tooth. Avocado provides a creamy base, while cocoa powder adds a hint of chocolate flavor.

Ingredients:

- 1 ripe avocado, peeled and pitted

- 1/2 cup low-fat milk (or lactose-free milk)

- 1/4 cup cocoa powder (optional)

- 1 tablespoon honey

Instructions:

1. In a blender, combine avocado, milk, cocoa powder (if using), and honey.

2. Blend until smooth and creamy.

3. Pour the mixture into popsicle molds.

4. Freeze for at least 4 hours, or until solid.

Nutritional Information (per serving):

- Calories: 200

- Protein: 2g

- Carbohydrates: 25g

- Fat: 10g

Part 3: Living Your Best Life with an Ileostomy

Chapter 9: Staying Active with an Ileostomy

Living with an ileostomy doesn't mean giving up on an active lifestyle. In fact, regular exercise can be incredibly beneficial for your overall health and well-being. It can improve your cardiovascular health, strengthen your muscles, and boost your mood. But with an ileostomy, there are a few additional considerations to keep in mind to ensure a safe and enjoyable workout experience.

Finding the Right Exercise Routine

The good news is that most forms of exercise are safe for people with ileostomies, with a few exceptions. Here are some tips for finding the right exercise routine for you:

- **Start Slowly:** If you're new to exercise, or haven't been active in a while, it's important to begin slowly and gradually increase the intensity and duration of your workouts. This will help your body adjust and reduce the risk of injury.

- **Listen to Your Body:** Pay attention to how your body feels during and after exercise. If you experience any pain, discomfort, or leakage from your pouch, stop the activity and consult your doctor.

- **Talk to Your Doctor:** Before starting a new exercise program, it's always a good idea to talk to your doctor. They can help you create a safe and effective routine that considers your individual needs and limitations.

- **Choose Activities You Enjoy:** You're more likely to stick with an exercise program if you enjoy the activities you choose. Explore different options such as walking, swimming, cycling, yoga, or dancing.

- **Consider Support Groups:** Joining an ileostomy support group can be a great way to connect with others who understand the challenges and benefits of living with an ostomy. You can share tips, advice, and motivation for staying active.

Activities to Avoid:

While most exercises are safe, there are a few that may not be suitable for people with ileostomies. These include:

- Contact sports with a high risk of collision (e.g., football, rugby)

- Heavy weightlifting that puts excessive strain on your abdominal muscles

Adapting Activities:

Many activities can be adapted for people with ileostomies. For example, you can wear a supportive ostomy belt during exercise to help keep your pouch secure. You can also modify exercises to avoid putting too much strain on your abdominal muscles.

Staying Hydrated During Exercise

Hydration is crucial for everyone, but especially important for people with ileostomies. Exercise can lead to fluid loss through sweat, which can dehydrate you and thicken your output. Here are some tips for staying hydrated during exercise:

- **Drink plenty of fluids before, during, and after your workout.** Aim to drink 16-20 ounces of water 2-3 hours before exercise, and then 4-8 ounces every 15-20 minutes during your workout.

- **Consider electrolyte drinks:** If you're sweating heavily, you may also benefit from electrolyte drinks that can help replenish lost electrolytes. Talk to your doctor about the best options for you.

- **Carry a water bottle with you:** Keep a water bottle handy during your workout so you can sip on fluids regularly.

- **Monitor your urine:** Pay attention to the color of your urine. Dark yellow urine is a sign of dehydration.

By following these tips, you can stay safe, hydrated, and enjoy the many benefits of exercise with an ileostomy. Remember, an active lifestyle is an important part of overall health and well-being, and it's definitely achievable with a little planning and adaptation.

Long-Term Ileostomy Care and Wellness

Living with an ileostomy is a lifelong journey, but it doesn't have to hold you back from living a full and healthy life. By following a few key practices, you can ensure your long-term well-being and embrace all that life has to offer.

Regular Doctor Visits and Checkups

Scheduling regular checkups with your doctor is essential for maintaining good health with an ileostomy. These visits allow your doctor to monitor your overall health, check your stoma and peristomal skin, and address any concerns you may have.

Here's what to expect during your doctor visits:

- **General health check:** Your doctor will likely check your blood pressure, weight, and temperature.

They may also ask about your overall health and well-being.

- **Stoma check:** Your doctor will examine your stoma to ensure it's healthy and functioning properly. They will also check the surrounding skin for any signs of irritation or infection.

- **Blood tests:** Your doctor may order blood tests to check your electrolyte levels, nutrient absorption, and overall health.

- **Open communication:** Don't hesitate to ask your doctor any questions you may have about your ileostomy, your health, or any concerns you experience.

Frequency of Checkups:

The frequency of your doctor visits will vary depending on your individual needs and health status. Typically, you can expect to see your doctor every 3-6 months in the first year after surgery, and then annually thereafter.

Maintaining a Healthy Weight

Maintaining a healthy weight is important for everyone, but it's especially crucial for people with ileostomies. A healthy weight can help reduce strain on your abdominal muscles, improve nutrient absorption, and lower your risk of developing other health problems.

Here are some tips for maintaining a healthy weight with an ileostomy:

- **Eat a balanced diet:** Focus on consuming a variety of nutritious foods from all food groups.

- **Manage portion sizes:** Pay attention to portion sizes and avoid overeating.

- **Stay active:** Regular exercise helps you maintain a healthy weight and overall well-being.

- **Talk to a registered dietitian:** A registered dietitian can help you create a personalized meal plan that meets your nutritional needs and supports a healthy weight.

Staying Positive and Embracing Life

An ileostomy can bring about emotional challenges. It's natural to feel overwhelmed, frustrated, or anxious at times. However, it's important to remember that you're not alone. There are many resources available to help you cope and adjust to life with an ileostomy.

Here are some tips for staying positive and embracing life:

- **Connect with others:** Join an ostomy support group or connect with others online who understand the challenges and triumphs of living with an ileostomy.

- **Focus on the positive:** Living with an ileostomy allows you to live a full and active life. Celebrate your milestones and achievements, big or small.

- **Practice relaxation techniques:** Techniques like meditation, yoga, or deep breathing can help manage stress and improve your overall well-being.

- **Seek professional help:** If you're struggling to cope emotionally, don't hesitate to seek professional help from a therapist or counselor.

Living with an ileostomy may require some adjustments, but with the right care and support, you can thrive and live a fulfilling life. Remember, the future is bright, and you have the power to create a healthy and happy future for yourself.

Sample Ileostomy Meal Plans for Different Needs:

Here are some sample meal plans tailored to address different needs:

- **General Ileostomy Meal Plan:** This plan provides a well-balanced foundation for most individuals.

    - Breakfast: Greek yogurt with berries and granola, scrambled eggs with whole-wheat toast

    - Lunch: Baked chicken breast with roasted vegetables and brown rice, tuna salad on whole-wheat bread with lettuce and tomato

    - Dinner: Salmon with steamed asparagus and quinoa, lentil soup with whole-grain bread

- Snacks: Apple slices with almond butter, carrot sticks with hummus, low-fibre banana bread

- **High-Calorie Meal Plan:** This plan is suitable for individuals who need to increase their calorie intake.

  - Breakfast: Oatmeal with protein powder, berries, and nuts, whole-wheat pancakes with fruit and maple syrup

  - Lunch: Chicken stir-fry with brown rice and vegetables, turkey burger on a whole-wheat bun with avocado and sweet potato fries

  - Dinner: Baked cod with mashed potatoes and steamed broccoli, lentil pasta with vegetables and cheese

  - Snacks: Trail mix with nuts, seeds, and dried fruit, high-protein yogurt with granola and banana slices

- **Low-Fibre Meal Plan:** This plan focuses on low-fibre foods to minimize digestive discomfort.

  o Breakfast: Scrambled eggs with cheese and spinach, white toast with mashed avocado

  o Lunch: Grilled chicken breast on a white bun with lettuce and tomato, baked potato with low-fat cheese

  o Dinner: Baked salmon with roasted asparagus and white rice, cream of chicken soup with crackers

  o Snacks: Ripe banana with peanut butter, applesauce with cinnamon

High-Protein Meal Plan: This plan focuses on protein-rich foods to support healing and muscle building.

- Breakfast: Greek yogurt with protein powder and berries
- Lunch: Grilled chicken breast with brown rice and steamed broccoli

- Dinner: Baked salmon with roasted sweet potato and asparagus

- Snacks: Cottage cheese with sliced cucumber, protein shake

Low-Lactose Ileostomy Meal Plan: This plan is suitable for individuals who experience lactose intolerance.

- Breakfast: Gluten-free oatmeal with almond milk and berries

- Lunch: Grilled turkey sandwich on gluten-free bread with lettuce and tomato

- Dinner: Baked cod with quinoa and roasted vegetables

- Snacks: Lactose-free yogurt with fruit, rice cakes with almond butter

Stoma Care Guide:

- **Cleaning:** Gently clean your stoma and surrounding skin with warm water and mild soap at least once a day, and more often if needed. Pat the area dry with a soft towel and allow it to air dry completely before applying a new pouch.

- **Pouch Application:** Measure your stoma to ensure a proper fit for the pouch. Apply the pouch to clean, dry skin, ensuring a good seal around the stoma. Empty the pouch when it is one-third to half full.

- **Skin Care:** Use a stoma powder or paste to protect the skin around your stoma from irritation caused by pouch adhesive. Apply barrier wipes or cream to address any skin concerns.

- **Signs of Infection:** Watch for signs of infection around your stoma, such as redness, swelling, or pus. If you experience any of these symptoms, contact your doctor immediately.

Ileostomy Diet Food Chart:

Food Group	Allowed Foods	Foods to Limit
Fruits	Ripe bananas, melons,	Raw fruits (except

	applesauce, canned fruit (except pineapple)	ripe bananas), prune juice, grape juice
Vegetables	Well-cooked, peeled vegetables (potatoes, carrots, zucchini), lettuce	Raw vegetables (except lettuce), corn
Starches	White bread, pasta, rice, bagels, crackers	Whole-wheat bread, brown rice, bran cereals
Proteins	Lean meats (chicken, turkey, fish), smooth nut butters, eggs (start with a small amount)	Fried meats, high-fat meats, beans, lentils
Dairy	Low-fat milk, lactose-free milk, yogurt, cheese	Whole milk, high-fat dairy products, milk with lactose (if intolerant)
Drinks	Water, decaf coffee/tea, sports drinks, rehydration drinks	Carbonated drinks, alcoholic drinks (in moderation)

Please note: This is a general guideline, and individual needs may vary. Always consult with your doctor or a registered dietitian for personalized dietary advice.

9 7 9 8 8 8 4 6 5 9 6 3 6